How To Best Cope With Cancer

317 Extremely Helpful Tips To Conquer A Cancer Diagnosis

ADAM COLTON

Published by BizMove
www.bizmove.com

317 Extremely Helpful Tips To Conquer A Cancer Diagnosis

If you've recently been diagnosed with cancer, you have had to deal with shock and even grief, Now it's time to become a fighter. Here are some tips to help you deal with your illness and continue to enjoy life.

1. If you are battling cancer, it can be helpful to join a support group for your type of cancer or cancer in general. Talking to others in your situation can help you feel less alone and give you a chance to make new friends. Mutual support can be very important on the journey to recovery.

2. Ask your doctor plenty of questions. If you have just received a cancer diagnosis, make sure to get as much basic information as you can. Find out the type, if it can be treated, what the treatment would be, and if the cancer is spreading. The more you know the better chance you will have.

3. If a loved one receives a diagnosis of cancer, make yourself available to them. It may be difficult for you, but they need someone to listen while they express their feelings. Be sensitive

about the opinions you provide; not everyone suffers from the same things or sees the outcome in the same manner, but that shouldn't matter.

4. Lower your odds of developing colon cancer by about 40 percent by being physically active. Regular exercise helps you stay in shape, maintain an appropriate weight, and avoid diseases associated with higher cancer risk, such as diabetes. Strive always to stay active.

5. Expressing your love for someone with cancer doesn't always have to be done vocally. You can simply be there for a person physically to assist them and to show your moral support. Some types of cancer are incredibly rough, and the patient might not be able to care for him or herself. Make sure you're there for them.

6. Decrease the amount of red (such as lamb, pork, and beef) and processed meats in your diet. Studies have shown that red meat can increase your chances of getting cancer. If you do buy red meat, make sure that it is lean meat. You don't have to remove red meat from your diet, just limit it.

7. Participating in treatments that help you battle cancer is the best thing that you can do, as

opposed to just sitting and waiting for physicians to treat you. Don't settle for sitting on the sidelines. Actions like these are counterproductive to the healing process.

8. One important thing to consider is using sealant on any wood structures that were built before 2005. These items were constructed with a wood that had arsenic pesticide on it. If you put a seal on them you can prevent exposure of children to cancer-causing chemicals.

9. Avoid anemia during cancer treatments by eating foods rich in iron such as liver, green leafy vegetables, molasses and lentils. These foods will boost your iron levels allowing oxygen rich blood to be carried throughout your body and facilitates chemotherapy.

10. Mood swings and other similar symptoms are natural for those suffering from cancer. Knowing this can help you prepare for what you will encounter if you or a loved one are suffering with cancer.

11. For cancer patients who are not satisfied with their current treatment, know that you can get a second opinion. Sometimes, another oncologist may know of treatment options that can help

you. If you are unsure where to go for treatment, you can look online for good cancer treatment centers in your area.

12. If you are not coping very well, or even if you are coping well, consider looking for a support group in your area. They will be able to listen and relate to what you are going through and you will likely find a good bit of comfort in being surrounded by others who are going or have been through the things that you are.

13. Do not be afraid to talk to your doctor about pain medication during your cancer treatments. There are so many options available today to help you manage the side effects from your treatment that you should not have to be uncomfortable. Also speak to your physician if you don't like the way a prescription is making you feel.

14. Keep up a healthy, active lifestyle. Eat healthy, nutritious foods and exercise when possible. Keeping active can help you cope better with treatment and lead to a longer life. Also be sure to get enough sleep, which will help alleviate some of the stress of cancer treatment and fend off fatigue.

15. Many complementary therapies now exist which can work in conjunction with traditional cancer treatments and help to rid your body of the disease more quickly. Try getting a massage, using aromatherapy, getting an acupuncture treatment, or engaging in a yoga class. These are all ways to help you relax during one of the most stressful times in your life.

16. To try and prevent cancer, make sure you are having checkups regularly. Learn how often you need to be checked for different cancers, such as breast, prostate, lung, colon, cervix and skin. Early detection of cancer greatly increases your chance for a cure and decreases your risk of dying from cancer.

17. To prevent cancer, try and eat a balanced diet that is thought to reduce cancer risks, especially colon cancer. This diet includes eating less than four ounces of red meat a day, avoiding processed meats like bologna, eating a variety of non-starchy fruits and vegetables and avoiding excessive amounts of sugar.

18. Reduce your level of stress, especially if you have been diagnosed with cancer. Stress alone has not been proven to be a contributing factor to cancer, but a stressful routine leads to many

unhealthy activities that can easily increase the risk of cancer or hinder your recovery. Keep your stress level low.

19. Carcinogens are substances that damage DNA. They are instrumental in starting and aiding in the growth of cancers. Things to stay away from that are carcinogenic are tobacco, asbestos, x-rays, the sun and exhaust fumes. Exposure to these substances causes cells to stop functioning in a normal way.

20. Alcohol consumption is the number one cause of liver cancer. Alcohol abuse over time can damage the liver in such a way that it can no longer function. Without a transplant, most liver cancers are fatal. Reduce your risk of liver cancer by cutting down your alcohol consumption or eliminating it completely.

21. You should continue to work even if you have been diagnosed with cancer. Cancer does not have to be a life stopper unless you let it. As long as you are still physically able to work, you should. It will keep your mind occupied and show you that you still have a great purpose.

22. Aside from talking to your close friends, family members, and your doctor, you should also try to

talk to other cancer patients. Those who have had first hand experience with cancer will know better than anyone else what you are going through and they can offer support and share experiences to help you through.

23. There are many different ways that people cope with cancer. Some of them good and some of them bad. Find a good way to cope with cancer. Some good coping methods include relaxation techniques, such as meditation, doing leisure activities or writing your feelings down in a journal.

24. Here is a preventative cancer tip that many people may not like: You should try to limit the amount of fatty meat and high fat dairy products you consume daily. These products can contain carcinogens that often accumulate in the food chain through animal fat, such as PCB and dioxins.

25. Be aware that the fruits and vegetables you buy may be contaminated. They often carry chemicals meant to kill insects, fungus, or bacteria. If you can't buy untreated organic vegetables and fruits, make sure to wash your produce thoroughly.

26. Some people are misinformed when it comes to cancer. Certain people believe that cancer can be transferred from person to person, while others think that they can no longer work. Address other people's concerns as honestly as you can, and don't be afraid to share your own feelings about what you're going through.

27. Unfortunately, some people will contract cancer due to their genes, even if they lead a healthy, active lifestyle. You may want to consider undergoing some type of counseling if your DNA increases your risks of getting cancer. Being prepared for what's possibly to come will help you deal with it when it arrives.

28. While laughter may not be able to cure cancer, it can certainly help a little. People call laughter the best medicine for a good reason. Cancer is a very serious illness, but don't allow an overly-serious ambiance to envelop you permanently. This may inhibit some of the humor and laughter that would normally be spontaneous. Appreciating the humor in life will help you to feel a little better both physically a mentally.

29. Simple carbohydrates can actually increase your risk of getting cancer, but complex carbs, like whole grains, will reduce your risk significantly.

The germ, bran and endosperm of the whole grains are very rich in fiber, vitamins and minerals and can help you to prevent cancer in your stomach, colon and other areas of the body.

30. Attend doctor's appointments with your friend or family member who has been diagnosed with cancer. These appointments often involve long waits and can be a stressful experience. Write down important information that the doctor provides about their treatment and prognosis; your friend may have difficulty remembering what was said later on.

31. Individuals with cancer like to know what to expect from their treatments and the disease itself. Help them find information by looking online, visiting the local cancer center and asking questions of medical professionals. The information you gather could be crucial in helping them stay focused and maintain a positive attitude.

32. Be mindful of your exposure to BPA. This synthetic estrogen is often found in canned goods, water bottles and other items. Research has shown that BPA has the potential to cause cancer, so try to eat more frozen foods and look for water bottles that are labeled as BPA free.

33. Be totally honest with your friends and family about your cancer. Remember that these people will want to support you, and that this is a time when you not only deserve, but need that support. Open and honest communication is what will serve all of you best at this time.

34. Some foods can reduce the risk of developing certain cancers. For example, tomatoes can protect against prostate cancer. Many studies have been produced showing the type of foods that help fight cancer.

35. One of the alternative treatments to cancer that you can add in addition to your doctors orders is a mind and body therapy. This therapy focuses on behavior, faith and emotions. The treatments can include hypnosis, biofeedback and counseling. These techniques will not cure cancer but can greatly change your attitude about it and give your emotional life a lift.

36. As soon as you are diagnosed with cancer, you need to contact your insurance company to see what is covered and what isn't. Treatment can be extremely expensive, so you will want to know what is covered and what is not. Once you have this information, you should sit down and

discuss it with your doctor. You two can then come up with a treatment plan that will work for you and your budget.

37. Battling cancer can be the biggest fight of your life. You need to be informed and in control of all the options you have. Don't be afraid to ask questions of your doctors, nurses and other medical caregivers. Research your type of cancer and empower yourself with knowledge. Arming yourself for battle can help you win the war!

38. There are many different ways that people cope with cancer. Some of them good and some of them bad. Find a good way to cope with cancer. Some good coping methods include relaxation techniques, such as meditation, doing leisure activities or writing your feelings down in a journal.

39. One of the most critical things you can do to cope with your cancer diagnosis is taking the time to think about your goals and what you want from life. Participate in activities that you enjoy; they will make you feel happy and hopeful. Spend time with the people you love and don't waste your energy on other things.

40. It is important to read the warning labels for many products. Many people do not realize that products they use every day contain carcinogens. When buying products, pay careful attention to the ingredients of the product, and even look for warning labels that may say that the product you intend to purchase may cause cancer.

41. While laughter may not be able to cure cancer, it can certainly help a little. People call laughter the best medicine for a good reason. Cancer is a very serious illness, but don't allow an overly-serious ambiance to envelop you permanently. This may inhibit some of the humor and laughter that would normally be spontaneous. Appreciating the humor in life will help you to feel a little better both physically a mentally.

42. Depression often causes health issues of its own, which can lead to problems treating the cancer. Depression makes it more likely that someone will stop fighting their cancer.

43. Be open and honest with others. If you need additional help to get through this difficult period in your life, bring the topic up gently with your loved ones. Give them a patient explanation of how they can assist you and why it's important to do so. Practice caution in this situation

though. Dealing with cancer can be a challenging time. Make sure you base it all on love. It is critical that you not have any regrets at this point.

44. Beating cancer may require a little bit of luck, but you cannot allow yourself to rely on being lucky in order to beat it. In other words, you should never really expect miracles or for some experimental treatment to instantly cure you. Luck may play a role, but you should focus on putting in the effort to defeat cancer.

45. Know the signs and symptoms of lung cancer, and those that aren't so easy to see. Lung cancer is such a fatal disease, due to the fact that signs and symptoms often mask themselves as other conditions until the disease has spread throughout the lungs and caused greater damage.

46. Get to know your breasts. It may seem kind of silly to feel your breasts on a regular basis, but if you take the time to learn how they should feel, you are going to be able to notice any changes if they should occur. This makes it much easier for you to know when there is a change so you can see your doctor immediately.

47. Look for makeup that has a good SPF rating. Many women are not going to leave the house without wearing makeup and you can make that very beneficial to your skin. If you take the time to find a good makeup that will protect your skin as it makes you look pretty, you will benefit a good bit.

48. Do not be afraid to talk to your doctor about pain medication during your cancer treatments. There are so many options available today to help you manage the side effects from your treatment that you should not have to be uncomfortable. Also speak to your physician if you don't like the way a prescription is making you feel.

49. Keep your job as long as your body will allow you to. You will find that if you continue to work that you will find more meaning in your life. That will give you a way to spend your days without thinking about your disease the entire time. You will keep your mind sharp and feel good doing it.

50. Watch out for cancer treatment scams. After being diagnosed with cancer, you may feel desperate to try any treatment you can find. However, you should be careful and fully

research any treatment method you are considering. If a cancer "cure" sounds too good to be true, it probably is. Discuss and research the treatment with a reputable doctor or government agency before deciding on any treatment.

51. Help prevent cancer by keeping physically fit. If your body is in good health, you will have a greater chance of avoiding the disease, or fighting it off if you do encounter it. You do not need to be an Olympic athlete- any exercise that gets your heart pounding is effective.

52. Cancer is a very depressing disease. Knowing this, one of the best things that you can do for a person who is diagnosed with cancer is to add humor to their day. Humor is known to be the best medicine. Also make sure to be sensitive to their feelings when making jokes.

53. When you first receive your cancer diagnosis, get as many facts as you can about it. Try to gather as much useful, basic information as you can about the type of cancer you have. What kind of cancer is it? Where is it? Has it spread? How will it be treated?

54. If you are not feeling well you should not get behind the wheel of a car when you are going through cancer treatment. Many people who are battling cancer feel weaker than they normally would and easily fall asleep. You would not want to risk your life by falling asleep behind the wheel.

55. To stand a chance of surviving cancer you have to be willing to put up a fight against it. If you give up emotionally, the cancer will have a greater chance of taking over your body and ultimately ceasing your existence here. You have to fight to beat cancer.

56. When facing cancer, you should remember to anticipate physical changes. Cancer and cancer treatments such as chemotherapy will cause your body to experience changes, such as hair loss. Keeping these changes in mind will help you prepare for them in advance and remove any chances of being surprised by them. Find a patient physician who is willing to spend time discussing these matters with you.

57. Following your cancer diagnosis, try to keep your life as normal as possible. You may need to make some changes, but a consistent routine will help you feel more like yourself. Since your plans

may need to be altered at the drop of a hat, take each day as it comes and enjoy it.

58. Think about how you are going to cope with the stress of your cancer diagnosis. Everyone handles things differently, but it is important to have a way to relax after a particularly difficult day. Research relaxation techniques, consider which friends and family members you can talk openly with, and keep a journal.

59. Working to reduce your exposure to radiation is one of the best ways you can prevent cancer. Now, the jury's still out on whether or not cell-phone usage puts you at a higher risk of things like brain tumors, but there is a direct link between cancer and radiation. So do what you can to avoid radiation.

60. Try to avoid alternative and holistic remedies alone to fight cancer if you have it. Steve Jobs is a great example of holistic remedies failing. Medical professionals insist that modern medicine and surgery would have saved his life. It can save your life too, if you have cancer. Don't replace modern medicine with voodoo.

61. Every person with cancer believes that they are above the five known stages of grief, but the best

thing you can do is to accept that you are susceptible to them. Giving in to your emotions now means that you can get the denial out of the way and reach the acceptance stage where you fight back against the disease.

62. There is no conceivable reason that you have to live with unbearable pain as a cancer sufferer, so make sure that you are getting the right pain medication. There are dozens of pain meds out there, and if the one you're taking isn't working well, make sure you tell your doctor that you need something different.

63. Always wear sunscreen. Taking this simple step can help reduce the risk of getting cancer from the sun. Try to stay in the shade as much as possible and also wear clothing and hats that will protect your skin. Apply sunscreen liberally and often to get the maximum amount of protection possible.

64. If you have been diagnosed with cancer, drink as much water as possible, ideally between eight and ten glasses every day. You will be taking quite a bit of medication, and water helps your kidneys handle everything that you are putting into your body. Water will also keep you hydrated.

65. To cut the risk of getting cancer it is recommended that you stay as active as possible. At least 30 minutes of exercise a day is encouraged as it has been found that being overweight can be linked to getting cancer. So find an exercise you enjoy and give it some of your time each and every day.

66. Know your family history. Once of the causes of skin cancer is genetics. If you have members in your family that have had skin cancer, you may be at more of a risk to get it as well. If you have inherited the traits of the high risk factor, you need to be additionally careful when in the sun.

67. Unlike non-treated clothing, UV clothing will help protect your skin from the sun's damaging rays. If you are unable to locate protective apparel from local stores, you should be able to find it from online retailers.

68. Beware of the sun even on cloud covered days. The harmful rays of the sun are still making their way through the clouds and to your skin. Keep sunscreen applied even if you do not feel the heat of the sunrays. They are still causing the damage that they would if there was not a cloud in the sky.

69. Watch out for cancer treatment scams. After being diagnosed with cancer, you may feel desperate to try any treatment you can find. However, you should be careful and fully research any treatment method you are considering. If a cancer "cure" sounds too good to be true, it probably is. Discuss and research the treatment with a reputable doctor or government agency before deciding on any treatment.

70. Dealing with a devastating disease like cancer can cause many fears about life and death. A good way to help yourself overcome these feelings is to become more spiritual! Studies show that people who engage in regular worship and prayer fare much better and live longer than those who don't.

71. When battling cancer it is important for you to try to find humor somewhere. Many people fall into depression while they are battling cancer and do not even realize it. It is understandable for someone to feel depressed about the diagnosis but fighting is what helps save lives. Humor can be a great way to put up a fight.

72. Sit down and go over your goals and priorities. A cancer diagnosis provides a good reason to re-evaluate and reflect on your life. Some things that were important may no longer be as important as they were before. Are there activities that you have been thinking of doing or people you haven't seen that you would like to?

73. Maintaining a healthy diet can help you to keep your energy levels up if you have cancer. This disease is very draining on you emotionally and physically. Keeping high levels of energy is imperative if you hope to fight and beat this disease. Higher levels of energy mean you can exercise more and work to get healthy.

74. It's important that you work hard to deal with your feelings and emotions if you or someone you know has cancer. This is going to be a very emotional time in ways you cannot possibly understand unless you've been through it, and unchecked emotions can destroy relationships permanently and lead to a world of regret.

75. A good tip to deal with cancer in general is to make sure you earn yourself some good karma points. Donating to cancer research and other cancer-specific charities helps you to feel good and will certainly help assist in the ongoing fight

against this brutal disease. And if karma is real, airing on its good side wouldn't hurt.

76. If you feel concerned, always seek the guidance of a physician. If you are too proud or scared to visit the doctor, you could be ignoring issues that exist and could get worse. If there is cancer present, it could spread and cause greater harm, which could be avoided if you seek the guidance of a health care professional you trust.

77. Purchase mouthwash. Cancer treatment, including chemotherapy, will often cause you to form painful mouth ulcers. Mouthwash will help prevent these from occurring over time. Invest in a soft toothbrush as well, as regular tooth care can also impact the formation of mouth ulcers. These items will give you the added benefit of having fresh breath each day!

78. It is important that females get a pap smear done at least once every two years. If you have a history of gynecological problems, you may want to have one every year. Pap smears detect cervical cancer and changes in their cervical cells, which if caught early, is very treatable.

79. Talk to your doctor about anti-nausea medications if you are going through

chemotherapy. Nausea is one of the most common, but unfortunate side effects of chemotherapy, but it can be treated with medications. Most insurance plans will cover these drugs, as it is needed to help a patient manage their side effects.

80. Tanning salons have been linked to a wide number of skin cancer cases. They have been said to be just as dangerous to the human body as arsenic and mustard gas. Stop using tanning beds and get your golden glow from a spray booth or a bottle of self tanner.

81. One of the best ways in order to ease someone that has been diagnosed with cancer is to consciously listen to what they say. Listening to someone might sound easy but it is harder than it looks. With that said, it is important to not interrupt and listen to what they have to say with not only your ears but with your eyes and body as well.

82. If you are undergoing chemotherapy, consider getting your hair cut short. There is a good chance that your hair is going to fall out from the treatment and there will be much less to lose if you cut it short. This will make it an easier transition for you in the case that it does fall out.

83. If you are having difficulty sleeping as a result of your cancer treatment, develop a sleep routine for yourself. Go to bed and get up at the same time each day. Stay away from caffeine and do not drink alcohol. Engage in quiet activities before bed. All of these techniques will help your body understand when it is time to go to sleep.

84. Keep a phone handy whenever you are home. If you need to have one installed in your bedroom, do it, otherwise take your cordless phone with you wherever you go in your home. You may need it for emergencies or you may find it to be a great social connection when you are bored.

85. Discuss what will happen in the future with relatives who have cancer. If you give them the feeling that you believe they'll survive it, they're more likely to believe it themselves. Talking about their future is a good technique to make them believe that you think they will be around.

86. If you are battling cancer, it can be helpful to join a support group for your type of cancer or cancer in general. Talking to others in your situation can help you feel less alone and give you a chance to make new friends. Mutual

support can be very important on the journey to recovery.

87. If you are diagnosed with cancer, then you should remember to try to find out everything you can from your doctor about your illness and its treatment. Ask questions that will tell you what kind of cancer you have, what stage it is in, if it is treatable, where it is located, how far it has spread, and more. This will not only give you ease of mind, but it will inform you on the best ways to treat your cancer.

88. You should surround yourself with loved ones when you are fighting cancer. They will be able to give you encouragement when you need it or just be there to support you through the tough times. It is important to know that you are loved and that you would be missed if you did not fight.

89. Make certain to study any relevant text you can about the particular cancer you, or someone close to you, has. Confidence is actually very important here.

90. Always consider that a doctor you like, might not be the right doctor to help you beat your cancer. Sometimes, you have to go the extra mile

and seek out a specialist in the field with more expertise than your current oncologist may have. It's all about getting better and experts can help make this happen.

91. Because they are so rich in glutathione, avocados are a great cancer-preventing food you can eat. The reason avocados work to prevent cancer is that their powerful antioxidants wage a war against the free radicals floating around in your body. Eliminating free radicals is how you work to eliminate cancer cells.

92. You might not typically have a fighting spirit, but if you have cancer you are going to need to find one quickly. If you do not realize what you're fighting for and cannot develop that all-important spirit, use the anger you're feeling to transform into motivation. Even Gandhi was able to lash out.

93. Drinking a lot of water is a great way to not only help with taking your cancer medications, but also to prevent cancer altogether. Ample water in your system is great for your kidneys and will help to prevent constipation. It also helps to keep you properly hydrated, in order to keep your cells healthy.

94. There are a host of services you can contact in order to receive help with day-to-day tasks as you fight your cancer. You can contact local churches and charities or find some type of local government assistance. You will find people who will help you by cleaning your home and handing other things if you don't have anyone to lean on.

95. You will not always feel like cooking as your strength begins to fade, so make sure you're keeping healthy prepared meals in your fridge and freezer. While you have the strength to do it, prepare healthy food in advance. This way, you only have to microwave something for a few minutes when you need to eat.

96. Individuals with cancer like to know what to expect from their treatments and the disease itself. Help them find information by looking online, visiting the local cancer center and asking questions of medical professionals. The information you gather could be crucial in helping them stay focused and maintain a positive attitude.

97. Make sure that you are up-to-date on your immunizations. Viral infections can have an impact on certain types of cancer so ask your doctor whether you have received all the

necessary immunizations. In particular find out whether you have the Hepatitis B and HPV immunizations; these can help prevent liver cancer and cervical cancer.

98. Get to know your breasts. It may seem kind of silly to feel your breasts on a regular basis, but if you take the time to learn how they should feel, you are going to be able to notice any changes if they should occur. This makes it much easier for you to know when there is a change so you can see your doctor immediately.

99. Wear a strong SPF protection sunscreen every day. This can help to reduce your risk of skin cancer. The sun emits damaging ultraviolet rays, but sunscreen can help to protect you from them. Look for a high quality sunscreen that contains both UVA and UVB protection for best results.

100. For cancer patients that are taking chemotherapy, beware of nail loss. This is a common side effect of chemotherapy that doctors may not tell you about. If your nails do happen to fall out, be sure to keep on eye on them for infection, which is something that needs immediate treatment.

101.   If you feel as if you cannot express your true feelings about your disease and the treatment for it to your family, look into a social worker that your treatment center may have for you to talk with. If the center does not have one there, you are sure to find one through the internet in your area.

102.   Alcohol consumption has no safe amount when it concerns the risk of cancer. With each cocktail or beer, you are proportionally increasing your risk for particular forms of cancer. Your throat, mouth, and esophagus are all more susceptible to cancer if you drink alcohol regularly. Limiting the amount of alcohol you drink can reduce your risk for these cancers.

103.   Chemotherapy can damage the body in many ways. One key to remaining healthy throughout your treatment is to keep your weight stable and your immune system strong. If you are losing weight, eat calorie-rich, sugar-free foods. Also use foods and vitamins to boost your immune system, such as vitamin C, garlic and tomatoes.

104.   Cancer patients have to deal with many discomforts while being treated for their disease. One irritating side effect of chemotherapy is mouth sores or sore, irritated throat caused by

chemotherapy and radiation treatments. One natural way to soothe these painful sores is to drink aloe vera juice. This can be found at any health food store.

105.   One of the best ways to avoid getting cancer is to avoid doing things which may cause cancer. Two of the biggest offenders when it comes to causing cancer are smoking and tanning beds. Staying away from these two things gives you a much better chance at being cancer free.

106.   Carcinogens are substances that damage DNA. They are instrumental in starting and aiding in the growth of cancers. Things to stay away from that are carcinogenic are tobacco, asbestos, x-rays, the sun and exhaust fumes. Exposure to these substances causes cells to stop functioning in a normal way.

107.   Aside from talking to your close friends, family members, and your doctor, you should also try to talk to other cancer patients. Those who have had first hand experience with cancer will know better than anyone else what you are going through and they can offer support and share experiences to help you through.

108.   Ask your doctor plenty of questions. If you have just received a cancer diagnosis, make sure to get as much basic information as you can. Find out the type, if it can be treated, what the treatment would be, and if the cancer is spreading. The more you know the better chance you will have.

109.   Switching out coffee for green tea can help you to prevent catching cancer. Coffee will not necessarily increase your risks, but if you need a caffeine boost, green tea is full of EGCG and polyphenols. These substances help prevent cancer in the colon, liver, prostate, breast, and other areas of the body.

110.   Numerous studies have been conducted on garlic and its many medicinal qualities, but one of garlic's best medical benefits is that it helps to eliminate the cancer-causing cells produced in the body. People who eat garlic are able to kill upwards of 139% more tumor cells in the body than people who do not eat it.

111.   Beating cancer may require a little bit of luck, but you cannot allow yourself to rely on being lucky in order to beat it. In other words, you should never really expect miracles or for some experimental treatment to instantly cure you.

Luck may play a role, but you should focus on putting in the effort to defeat cancer.

112.   If you wear makeup, use products that do not contain chemicals that have been linked to cancer. There are websites online that can help you look up your favorite products to see what they have in them. Avoid products that contain ingredients with "peg" or "eth" as part of their name.

113.   If you are taking medication for cancer, it is important to always eat three meals a day. Even if you are not feeling very well, try to eat a little something. When your stomach is empty, you are more likely to experience nausea and other symptoms from your treatment. Foods like rice, bread, potatoes and fruits are all good food choices.

114.   Know your family history so you know if you are at risk of getting breast cancer. If you have family members who have had it before reaching menopause, be sure to tell your doctor. You are going to be at a higher risk of developing the cancer as well, and your doctor will want to keep a close eye on you.

115.   Limit the amount of red meats, and especially processed meats, in your diet. A healthy diet is linked to reduced risks of cancer. Eating a heavy amount of red, processed meats will increase the fat content of your diet. The processing in particular exposes you to some potentially harmful chemicals and preservatives. All of these things can be high risk factors for cancer.

116.   There are many types of clothing that aren't going to keep the sun from damaging your skin. If you are unable to locate protective apparel from local stores, you should be able to find it from online retailers.

117.   If you must be outside during the peak sun hours, try to stay in the shade as much as possible. Put up a canopy or just stay under a tree to avoid getting hit by direct sunlight. You will still get sun exposure, but you will not be as exposed to the harmful rays that can lead to cancer.

118.   Eating the right foods and exercising frequently can actually help to prevent cancer. By not exercising or by eating the wrong foods, you are increasing your risk of becoming obese. Obesity is a common cause of cancer and is

something that can easily be prevented. Try eating a diet full of fruits and vegetables.

119.   Once diagnosed with cancer, except the fact that your life is going to change forever. Adopt the attitude that you are now a fighter. If you go into the treatment with a positive thought process, you are surly going to be able to fight it with higher spirits and see better results that if you were ready to give up.

120.   If you have a friend or loved one suffering from cancer, there are many ways to show your love and support. One way is to accompany the person to doctor appointments and chemotherapy or radiation treatments. Cancer can be a lonely disease, and having a supportive partner can do wonders to lift the spirits of the one fighting it.

121.   When coping with cancer, you need to seek support from your friends and family. Many people do not realize that their loved ones want to be there to support them through the rough journey and that they will do anything to help the cancer patient feel more relaxed, comfortable, and loved.

122.   You should read books about cancer survivors when you are coping with cancer because it may help to give you inspiration. Reading inspirational books about survivors is a great way to give yourself the mental boost that is needed when you are feeling worried, stressed or depressed about your cancer.

123.   Aside from talking to your close friends, family members, and your doctor, you should also try to talk to other cancer patients. Those who have had first hand experience with cancer will know better than anyone else what you are going through and they can offer support and share experiences to help you through.

124.   People who suspect they may have cancer should rush to the doctor right away to get properly diagnosed. The earlier the cancer is caught in the body, the better your odds are of beating this terrible disease and living a normal life. Early stages of cancer can be defeated with therapy and/or surgery.

125.   Maintaining a healthy diet can help you to keep your energy levels up if you have cancer. This disease is very draining on you emotionally and physically. Keeping high levels of energy is imperative if you hope to fight and beat this

disease. Higher levels of energy mean you can exercise more and work to get healthy.

126.   Switching out coffee for green tea can help you to prevent catching cancer. Coffee will not necessarily increase your risks, but if you need a caffeine boost, green tea is full of EGCG and polyphenols. These substances help prevent cancer in the colon, liver, prostate, breast, and other areas of the body.

127.   Heart-healthy diets always suggest limiting the ingestion of red meat, and it should be the same for cancer-preventing diets. Always make sure you're not eating more than 11 ounces of red meat per week. The fat and cholesterol within red meat can increase your odds of contracting cancer, so take it easy on the meat.

128.   The life you had before cancer may seem like a distant memory as the battle wages on, but always cling to your past to remind yourself of what you have to look forward to in the future. Keep old pictures and old videos around to remind yourself that cancer is not all there is in life for you. A positive view of the future is good for for your health.

129.   Drinking a lot of water is a great way to not only help with taking your cancer medications, but also to prevent cancer altogether. Ample water in your system is great for your kidneys and will help to prevent constipation. It also helps to keep you properly hydrated, in order to keep your cells healthy.

130.   Keeping your mouth clean while you're experiencing chemotherapy is a must if you hope to prevent against mouth ulcers and even tooth loss. Failing to properly care for your mouth will cause cells inside of your mouth to rapidly divide and essentially tear up your mouth. Regular mouth wash can prevent this.

131.   Take every available opportunity to laugh and have a good time. Someone with cancer still needs to smile and enjoy life; your mood can be infectious, so stay positive and try to lighten the atmosphere. However, there will also be times that your friend needs to cry or feel sad, so it is important to also be respectful of that.

132.   Purchase mouthwash. Cancer treatment, including chemotherapy, will often cause you to form painful mouth ulcers. Mouthwash will help prevent these from occurring over time. Invest in a soft toothbrush as well, as regular tooth care

can also impact the formation of mouth ulcers. These items will give you the added benefit of having fresh breath each day!

133.   For people with moles on their bodies, be sure to always check for any changes, including an increase in size, a color change, or a change in shape. If you notice any of these changes, be sure to see a dermatologist immediately, as this could be a sign of skin cancer.

134.   If you are a cancer patient who enjoys getting facials, be sure to tell your aesthetician that you are receiving treatments. Although gentle exfoliant are okay for treating the dry skin that chemotherapy may cause, other ingredients in a facial, such as acidic products and peeling ingredients, may not be safe.

135.   If you are not coping very well, or even if you are coping well, consider looking for a support group in your area. They will be able to listen and relate to what you are going through and you will likely find a good bit of comfort in being surrounded by others who are going or have been through the things that you are.

136.   Did you know that consuming large amounts of sugar can actually make your cancer grow

more quickly? Cancer cells survive on sugar, so taking sugar out of your daily diet can help eliminate cancer cells. Although this tactic cannot eliminate the cancer on its own, it could be used with other kinds of therapies to combat cancer.

137.   If you are a woman, and breast cancer worries you. Then it is best to have been regular scheduled mammograms to make sure you are cancer free. Breast cancer is easily treated, and often successfully treated as long it's caught before the usual time by scheduling a routine mammogram you enable yourself to find out early enough to make a difference

138.   Do not isolate yourself from friends and family if you are diagnosed with cancer. Sometimes, people will become depressed and close up if they find out they have cancer. The emotional support from others will give you strength and a renewed energy to fight. You may be able to get useful advice from others who have experienced cancer as well.

139.   Beans are incredibly good for your heart, but they're also essential in preventing cancer, especially colon cancer. The amount of fiber contained in beans and legumes will help to rid

the body of free radicals via the fiber and also the saponins, phytic acid and protease inhibitors contained within the beans.

140.   Be open about how you are feeling, both physically and emotionally, and keep the lines of communication open. If you feel that your loved ones aren't being very supportive, bring up the topic in a non-aggressive but serious way. Kindly explain to them what they can do to help you. Caution is needed, though! These are very trying circumstances. The basis should always be love. Do not have any regrets!

141.   Try limiting fat in your diet. By decreasing the amount of fat, you will lower your cancer risk. Avoid frying, especially deep frying. There are alternatives to frying such as baking, roasting, broiling, and steaming. Try to buy the low or non fat versions of your favorite foods, like milk and yogurt.

142.   Always be ready for a battle. You are indisputably in a fierce battle to stay alive, and remaining strong and steadfast, fully prepared for the long haul, will place you at best advantage for eventual triumph.

143.   Maintain an honest approach when dealing with someone who has cancer. Your friend or family member may have to make difficult decisions about their future needs, and they need to know what to expect. It is also important to share as much information as possible with other family members, so they can begin dealing with their own emotions.

144.   In an effort to prevent cancer - stay away from tobacco products! This includes smoking and chewing tobacco. These items have been shown to increase the likelihood that you will develop lung, bladder, cervical, oral, and pancreatic as well as kidney cancer. Avoiding them will not only help reduce your risk of cancer, it will help you lead a healthier lifestyle overall.

145.   Beware of the sun even on cloud covered days. The harmful rays of the sun are still making their way through the clouds and to your skin. Keep sunscreen applied even if you do not feel the heat of the sunrays. They are still causing the damage that they would if there was not a cloud in the sky.

146.   Put traveling off for now! If you are receiving chemotherapy or radiation treatment

for cancer, it may be wise not to travel. First and foremost, you do not want to skip any treatments! Also, your immune system is weak and traveling - increases your risk of getting sick or getting an infection - which can cause major problems!

147.   Beware that breast cancer can occur in women of all ages. Many women think that because they are in their twenties or thirties that they cannot get breast cancer, therefore, they ignore symptoms, like lumps in their breasts. If you feel anything suspicious, be sure to let your doctor know.

148.   Keep up a healthy, active lifestyle. Eat healthy, nutritious foods and exercise when possible. Keeping active can help you cope better with treatment and lead to a longer life. Also be sure to get enough sleep, which will help alleviate some of the stress of cancer treatment and fend off fatigue.

149.   If you have beaten cancer, it is still important that you regularly see your doctor for checkups. Even it may be gone now, certain cancers can come back or they can begin in other parts of the body. If you notice any new symptoms, be sure to see your doctor right away.

150.   Your body and mind are going to react to the many treatments that you are going to go through. You need to stay on top of how you are processing things in your mind so that if things are slipping, you can let your caregiver know as soon as possible.

151.   A great way to cope with a cancer diagnosis is to keep an open dialogue with everyone in your life. Make sure you have a doctor you're comfortable with, so you can ask clarifying questions without feeling intimidated. Bring family members along so they will understand what is going on, and you can later talk openly about the appointment.

152.   The absolute best way to get a leg up in the battle against cancer is early detection. Be prepared to make appointments for screening tests, which will let you know if you have cancer before any symptoms appear. For testes and breast cancer, do self-exams monthly so that you may determine anything unusual.

153.   It is quite normal for cancer patients to feel unattractive. Self-esteem is at an all-time low and nothing seems to be right. This is a great time to pamper yourself! When you are feeling well

enough, take a friend and go out to lunch. Get your nails done, or shop for a new outfit. Doing normal, everyday activities can make you feel like part of life again and change your whole attitude!

154.   It's important to take detection and the possibility of early treatment, seriously, when thinking about cancer. Learn how to self-examine yourself for cancers of the skin, colon, prostate, cervix and breast. Be sure to perform checks regularly so that you can start fighting early and give yourself the best chance possible.

155.   When facing cancer, you should remember to anticipate physical changes. Cancer and cancer treatments such as chemotherapy will cause your body to experience changes, such as hair loss. Keeping these changes in mind will help you prepare for them in advance and remove any chances of being surprised by them. Find a patient physician who is willing to spend time discussing these matters with you.

156.   Lung cancer is one of the most deadly cancers. It is very difficult to treat, but scientists have discovered that diet may play a major role in reducing the incidence of this type of cancer. A diet low in fat and high in fruits, tomatoes and green vegetables all can reduce the risk. In fact,

studies show that apples can reduce the risk of lung cancer by as much as 50 per cent!

157.   Recognize intellectually that your physical appearance will probably change after a cancer diagnosis. If you go into treatment anticipating that you will eventually look different, you will have a much better attitude when those changes actually take place. Talk to your doctor about what to expect as you prepare to begin your journey.

158.   Don't be afraid to ask for help from family and friends. Pride may keep you from requesting aid, however, you may become weak when undergoing treatment. Your loved ones can do small chores and errands like shopping or cleaning the home. Just doing small tasks can ease your burden.

159.   Prepare yourself and your family for the worst if you have cancer. You always want to remain optimistic, but you also have to be realistic. You should have everything planned should the worst happen and you not recover. It's depressing and incredibly sad, but it is a possible truth you are facing and it needs to be dealt with.

160.   If you have been diagnosed with cancer, you should be willing to take help from wherever it may come. Help could come from family and friends, your place of worship, or even the community overall. You can find help out there; be sure to take it. You might not be able to work with cancer and the emotional toll may be too much to handle alone.

161.   Whether you are healthy or stricken with cancer, the worst thing you can do is smoke. Do not smoke under any circumstances. Smoking is a known cause of cancer with 100s of carcinogens in a cigarette. Not only that, smoking can exacerbate cancer and its symptoms and make it worse.

162.   It's important that you stick to a regular eating schedule when you're fighting cancer. The food may want to exit the same way it entered due to your chemo, but you cannot afford to skip meals here. Losing strength means that you are losing the fight. Work to stay strong so that you can beat the cancer.

163.   When you are dealing with cancer, you want to have a sufficient support group. This support group can get you through the worst of times and even the best of times, offering the support

that is needed and the motivation you need to continue with your treatment and therapy measures.

164.   Exclusively breastfeeding your baby for at least six months can provide him with valuable health protection later in life, including cancer protection. Scientists are not one hundred percent sure why this can protect your child, but it appears that the healthy immunity boosters they receive from breast milk can have a lifelong effect.

165.   Beware of mouth sores if you are going through chemotherapy. It can be one of many unpleasant side effects. Even so, they can be prevented or treated. Sucking on-ice chips, sucking on hard candies and drinking plenty of fluids can all help prevent mouth sores. Be sure to visit your dentist for checkups as well.

166.   Make time to go outside and enjoy the fresh air. Your cancer treatments may make it impossible for you to exercise, but spending time outside will help you feel refreshed and rejuvenated. If you can walk or participate in a light jog do that as well. Exercise is important to the healing process.

167.   To prevent cancer, try and eat a balanced diet that is thought to reduce cancer risks, especially colon cancer. This diet includes eating less than four ounces of red meat a day, avoiding processed meats like bologna, eating a variety of non-starchy fruits and vegetables and avoiding excessive amounts of sugar.

168.   If you are battling cancer, it can be helpful to join a support group for your type of cancer or cancer in general. Talking to others in your situation can help you feel less alone and give you a chance to make new friends. Mutual support can be very important on the journey to recovery.

169.   Laughter is a great way to cope with cancer. Many people find it hard to find humor in their life after they have been diagnosed with cancer but if you have humor in your life, you will feel stronger overall. The more you laugh the better chance you have of fighting the cancer.

170.   Older adults are at higher risk for developing certain types of cancer. Approximately 75% of cancers are diagnosed in people aged 55 and older. As the risk rises, so does the importance of staying healthy and physically fit. Regular doctor visits, normal body weight, a healthy diet,

self-exams and cancer screening tests can all help to reduce the risk.

171.   Do not be afraid to ask for help following your cancer diagnosis. Friends and family members often want to do everything they can to assist you; let them pick up items from the grocery store, take you to appointments or make you dinner. It makes them feel good to do something for you, and it makes your life a little easier.

172.   If you know someone with a diagnosis of cancer, give them the opportunity to talk to you. When someone has been diagnosed with this frightening disease, they have a great need to be heard. Make sure not to give your personal opinions or interrupt; this time is for them.

173.   Depression affects your physical health as well as your state of mind; it may even accelerate cancer growth. They might just give in.

174.   They say that eating an apple a day will keep the doctor away, but eating an onion a day can actually keep cancer at bay. Because of the large amount of antioxidants founds in onions, eating them regularly can help to eliminate free radicals

from your body and thus help you to prevent contracting cancer.

175.   Heart-healthy diets always suggest limiting the ingestion of red meat, and it should be the same for cancer-preventing diets. Always make sure you're not eating more than 11 ounces of red meat per week. The fat and cholesterol within red meat can increase your odds of contracting cancer, so take it easy on the meat.

176.   Don't let the fight frighten you. You'll maximize your chances for victory over the cancer if you go into it with a fighting attitude.

177.   Do not let someone fool you by telling you that alcohol helps prevent and fight against cancer. The properties of red wine have led to an increase in popularity as an anti-cancer food. Drinking too much alcohol will increase the risk of cancer.

178.   Drink pomegranate juice on a regular basis. Have at least 16 ounces a day for it to be effective. Pomegranate juice has a great deal of anti-cancer agents including polyphenols, isoflavones and ellagic acid. Several studies have shown a significant decrease in cancer risk and

some studies even imply that it can slow cancer down.

179.   You should know what some cancer symptoms are and how you can know when you're possibly at risk. Learning how to recognize signs and symptoms of cancer is the best way to prevent it.

180.   Tanning salons have been linked to a wide number of skin cancer cases. They have been said to be just as dangerous to the human body as arsenic and mustard gas. Stop using tanning beds and get your golden glow from a spray booth or a bottle of self tanner.

181.   You may feel that you are going to be fine to take yourself to your appointments for treatment but do not hesitate to ask a loved one for help getting there. You will find your loved ones will do just about anything to help you through this difficult time including driving you to your appointments.

182.   If you are the parent of a child who has leukemia or another kind of cancer, it is important that you put on a brave front. Your child feeds off of your energy and by letting them see you sad, they are going to feel helpless.

However, it is still important that you try to explain to them what is going on.

183.   Stay organized. You are going to have many appointments to go to and have to keep track of many different dates. Get a calendar and use it to keep track of things that are important. You can even log how you have felt on different days so you can let your doctor in on your progress.

184.   To prevent cancer, try and eat a balanced diet that is thought to reduce cancer risks, especially colon cancer. This diet includes eating less than four ounces of red meat a day, avoiding processed meats like bologna, eating a variety of non-starchy fruits and vegetables and avoiding excessive amounts of sugar.

185.   If you have a loved one that is experiencing cancer, a good way to encourage them is to go with them on their appointments. Attending appointments will let them know that you love and care for them. Hospitals and clinics can be frightening to some people, and waiting long hours can be really boring. With that said, having a companion is really a big deal.

186.   There are many different ways that people cope with cancer. Some of them good and some

of them bad. Find a good way to cope with cancer. Some good coping methods include relaxation techniques, such as meditation, doing leisure activities or writing your feelings down in a journal.

187.   Sit down and go over your goals and priorities. A cancer diagnosis provides a good reason to re-evaluate and reflect on your life. Some things that were important may no longer be as important as they were before. Are there activities that you have been thinking of doing or people you haven't seen that you would like to?

188.   Don't change your life drastically. It may be better if you try to maintain your lifestyle as it was while introducing necessary modifications. A big change can increase your stress level and confuse the people around you. Take every day at a time and make changes to your life as is needed.

189.   Here is one of the most important tips for cancer prevention in existence. Avoid BPA at all costs. BPA, also known as Bisphenol A, is a synthetic estrogen. It is found in hard plastics such as those that are used for water bottles and the interior of canned foods. BPA has been

linked to cancer in many cases. In order to avoid
BPA, use products that do not contain it.

190.   Someone with cancer is going to want and
need their time alone, so you have to know when
to back off and to give a person some space.
Having pride is important to everyone and
sometimes, people do not want you to see them
so vulnerable. Respect their request for privacy
or you might be pushed away completely.

191.   A great way for cancer survivors to deal and
to know what lies ahead is to network with other
survivors. There are plenty of cancer survivors in
the world, thankfully, and they meet up at
support groups and even on internet forums, so
you can always keep in contact with other
survivors.

192.   Be prepared to make new "friends" when
you have cancer; i.e. people you have to let into
your life with open arms. As a cancer patient,
you're going to be introduced to nurses, chemo
specialists, oncologists and many other medical
professionals. It is impossible to go it alone, so
welcome these new people into your life with
open arms.

193.   What you expect to have happen, and what actually happens, are two different things. Value all of the support you receive.

194.   Cancer doesn't have to take root in your brain in order to play tricks on your mind, so always remember to keep fantasy and reality separated from one another. You will begin to feel as if you're sleepwalking and dreaming while you're awake during your bout with chemo. Keep your mind focused and simply ignore the "weirdness."□

195.   For cancer patients in an extreme amount of pain, you may want to consider acupuncture. One of the many positive results of acupuncture is that it helps to ease pain. There are even certain insurance companies who will cover acupuncture, if it is being used to manage pain from cancer.

196.   Avoiding getting cancer is by far the easiest way to beat it. Skin cancer is one of the most preventable cancers. Simply using a good sunscreen, and protecting your skin from prolonged sun exposure is extremely effective in preventing melanomas.

197.   One way to help prevent cancer is to stay thin without becoming underweight. Being overweight leaves your body and its organs susceptible to many diseases especially certain cancers. Maintain a healthy weight and incorporate diet and exercise into your daily routine to stay healthy and cancer free.

198.   Some cancer treatments have been known to cause diarrhea. If that's the case in your treatment, consider eliminating coffee from your diet. Although coffee can help you stay alert, it contributes to diarrhea. The less caffeine you take in, the less diarrhea you'll experience.

199.   Find a great support system if you are diagnosed with cancer. This can be from family and friends or through organizations dedicated to helping a person through this traumatic process. If you find that some people in your life are toxic rather than helpful, it is best to limit the time you spend with those people.

200.   Cancer can take a toll on the patient as well as those close to one with cancer. Keeping a healthy balance is important. When you feel up to it, surround yourself with friends and family and activities that you enjoy. This will boost your mood and the mood of others around you.

People react to cancer in many different ways, and it is important to try to keep your spirits up.

201.   Install a panic button of some kind in your bathroom. You are going to need to shower regularly and there are going to be days that you are weaker than others. If you find yourself in the position that you need help, you need to be able to alert someone that you need that help.

202.   Consider adding selenium to your diet to help fight cancer. Selenium has proven beneficial in many laboratory tests. The positive effects can especially be seen when it comes to fighting prostate cancer. Consult your doctor before adding this supplement though, as it is counterproductive Cancer is a word that most people dread hearing all their lives. Many don't even get regular check-ups for fear of this word. But by taking advantage of the latest cancer screening tests, such as mammography and colonoscopy, you will give yourself the best odds of never having to hear the dreaded "C" word!

203.   With cancer, early detection is important and will increase the chance of cure. Talk with your doctor and set up regular times for screenings to best eliminate the chance for early cancer growth to get out of hand without treatment. Self

examinations once a month can help you to detect any early signs of breast or testicular cancer.

204.   Maintain a healthy weight and diet and get plenty of exercise. Not only can it help you feel great everyday, but it can lower cancer risks too. Follow a healthy diet routine, like nourishing yourself with vegetables and fruits, as well as keeping hydrated with water, while you exercise for at least half a hour every day may reduce your chances of obtaining cancer.

205.   Lung cancer is one of the most deadly cancers. It is very difficult to treat, but scientists have discovered that diet may play a major role in reducing the incidence of this type of cancer. A diet low in fat and high in fruits, tomatoes and green vegetables all can reduce the risk. In fact, studies show that apples can reduce the risk of lung cancer by as much as 50 per cent!

206.   Expressing your love for someone with cancer doesn't always have to be done vocally. You can simply be there for a person physically to assist them and to show your moral support. Some types of cancer are incredibly rough, and the patient might not be able to care for him or herself. Make sure you're there for them.

207.   Many, many people have gone through cancer, even as survivors themselves or through someone they love. So you can find plenty of moral support via live groups, online chat rooms and forums, and other areas. You can even start a group and speak with people who are going through the same thing you are.

208.   There is always a chance that a mammogram won't be able to spot any tumor, so a manual breast inspection is in order if you want thorough results. A skilled mammogram technician should also be skilled at giving a manual exam and also skilled in showing you how to give yourself a breast exam.

209.   When you're battling cancer, it's important to try to sleep without the aid of medications and alcohol. Falling asleep naturally, and for a long time if possible, will help your body's cells to regenerate and become healthier. When you're tired, try to give into the sleep, rather than fight it.

210.   Fresh air is definitely underrated but certainly helpful as you're attempting to beat cancer. Enjoying the sunshine and the breeze can be very calm, relaxing and refreshing. And if you

can walk around outside, you're also receiving the added benefit of exercise. Get out in the open air if you are able.

211.   You should always seek second opinions, even if you believe your oncologist is the best in his or her field. It's only an opinion you're seeking; you never know when someone made a mistake or failed to mention a possible treatment option to you. Getting multiple opinions will simply give you multiple sources of information.

212.   When you are first diagnosed with cancer, you should immediately make an appointment with your dentist. When making your appointment, inform the receptionist of your diagnosis so they can get you in quickly. Treatment can sometimes affect your oral health. Therefore, before starting any treatment plan it is necessary to have a dental cleaning and any necessary dental work done.

213.   Many people suffering with cancer also have post-traumatic stress disorder, commonly known as PTSD. If you notice that you have any of the symptoms of PTSD, you should immediately get help from a professional. Symptoms of PTSD include aversion to people or places, flashbacks

of events, irrational fears, and changes in your
sleep patterns.

214.   If you are one of the many women that has
dense breast tissue, find a mammogram facility
that works with digital imagery. Digital scans will
do a much better job at detecting cancer in the
women with dense breast tissue than the
traditional film would. It will provide your
doctor with a clearer image and make it easier to
read the images.

215.   It is important for cancer patients to drink
plenty of water, especially if they are receiving
chemotherapy. A cancer patient's immune
system is low and it is important to stay
hydrated. Becoming dehydrated can cause other
complications that could land you in the hospital.
Try to stay away from soda and sugary drinks.

216.   The best way to beat cancer is not to get it in
the first place. Skin cancer can be prevented by
avoiding overexposure to the sun. In any
instance when you will be spending a long period
in the sun, apply an adequate sunscreen product
to all areas of your skin.

217.   Avoid using pesticides with arsenic! It may
help your gardens to flourish, but it is can do

extreme damage to your body. Exposure over time can lead to skin cancer. There are many other kinds of pesticides that you can use - that will do the same job for your garden - but without the damage to you.

218.   Don't take part in dangerous, risky behaviors. Riskier activities can make it much more likely that an individual can develop an infection, increasing the likelihood of cancer in the future. Don't share needles and always practice safe sex when involved in intimate relations.

219.   Battling cancer can be the biggest fight of your life. You need to be informed and in control of all the options you have. Don't be afraid to ask questions of your doctors, nurses and other medical caregivers. Research your type of cancer and empower yourself with knowledge. Arming yourself for battle can help you win the war!

220.   When battling cancer it is important for you to try to find humor somewhere. Many people fall into depression while they are battling cancer and do not even realize it. It is understandable for someone to feel depressed about the

diagnosis but fighting is what helps save lives. Humor can be a great way to put up a fight.

221.   It is important to eat well when you are battling any form of cancer. When you are receiving treatment, you may feel nauseous or weak. There are certain foods that you can eat to feel less ill or to feel stronger throughout the day. You need to learn what those foods are and eat them on a regular basis.

222.   If you have cancer or if someone you love has the disease, one of the first things you should do is work to deal with your own feelings on the matter. Do not allow for any negative feelings to bleed over into someone else's life. Face those fears head on and work on keeping those emotions at bay.

223.   Spirituality plays an important role in the fight against cancer. Now, you do not have to believe in any higher power per se, but there is plenty of documented evidence that a person's belief in something greater than themselves can instill the confidence necessary to fight cancer until it's defeated.

224.   Women hoping to prevent breast cancer should choose their physicians wisely. Always

make sure to visit an expert in mammography. A start-up clinic or a medical professional straight out of school may not be your best option. Find someone with plenty of experience in the field to improve your chances of catching signs of cancer early.

225.   A good tip to deal with cancer in general is to make sure you earn yourself some good karma points. Donating to cancer research and other cancer-specific charities helps you to feel good and will certainly help assist in the ongoing fight against this brutal disease. And if karma is real, airing on its good side wouldn't hurt.

226.   We all know that carrots are good for your eyesight, but this root vegetable is also essential in fighting against cancer. It's amazing how simple things from nature can help to prevent such a disease; and with the beta-carotene and falcarinol found in carrots, throat, stomach, lung, bladder and other types of cancers can be prevented.

227.   The life you had before cancer may seem like a distant memory as the battle wages on, but always cling to your past to remind yourself of what you have to look forward to in the future. Keep old pictures and old videos around to

remind yourself that cancer is not all there is in life for you. A positive view of the future is good for for your health.

228.   Try to tone down the amount of time you spend in the sun. People underestimate the amount of risk involved with excessive sun exposure. Spending increased time in the sun increases your risk of skin cancer. Make sure to use a high SPF sunscreen, cover unprotected skin and cover your head with a hat.

229.   For women, a mammogram is a great way to prevent breast cancer. A regularly schedule mammogram allows doctors to detect any lumps in breast tissue. Lumps in the breast tissue are a possible sign of breast cancer. Self breast exams should also be performed by women at home.

230.   If you live alone, try to stock up on meals when you feel well. Cook up a large batch of chicken or soup and freeze it. Since there will probably be days when your cancer treatment leaves you feeling a little weak, it will be very helpful to be able to quickly heat up a meal and relax.

231.   Find some kind of humor in your days. Laughter is good for the mind, body and spirit. If

you can find at least one thing to laugh about each hour of every day, you are going to benefit from the chemicals it will release in your body and the uplifting it will do for your spirit.

232.   Talk with other survivors. A cancer diagnosis can be overwhelming and it can feel like no one understands what it is like. Talk with family members or friends who has gone through it themselves or join a support group. From them, you can get insight into what treatment will be like and how to handle your diagnosis.

233.   Start a journal. Sit down each evening and spend a few times expressing your thoughts and feelings in a private journal. Write poetry if it helps you to get these feelings out. Letting them out, even if nobody else knows them, is going to help you cope with this tough situation.

234.   One of the best ways in order to ease someone that has been diagnosed with cancer is to consciously listen to what they say. Listening to someone might sound easy but it is harder than it looks. With that said, it is important to not interrupt and listen to what they have to say with not only your ears but with your eyes and body as well.

235.   Vitamin C is a natural enemy to cancer. Vitamin C tricks tumors into thinking they are getting sugar, which cancer cells feed on. When cancer uses vitamin C as an energy source, The vitamin begins to destroy cancer cells, thus slowing down their multiplication. In turn, the growth of tumors can be slowed down.

236.   Sugar can contribute to cancer growing in your body, so reduce your consumption of this product. Cancer cells love sugar, so getting rid of the sugar you consume can help stop cancer cell growth. While this tactic on its own may not eliminate the cancer, it can be used in conjunction with other therapy to combat cancer.

237.   One of the most important tips to remember after being diagnosed with cancer is to maintain a healthy life style. Maintaining a healthy lifestyle will give you more energy, which you will need during the treatment process. A healthy lifestyle consists of eating healthy foods and doing regular exercise.

238.   If you have cancer or if someone you love has the disease, one of the first things you should do is work to deal with your own feelings on the matter. Do not allow for any negative feelings to

bleed over into someone else's life. Face those fears head on and work on keeping those emotions at bay.

239.   As a cancer survivor, you should be making plans to permanently monitor the long-term effects of the treatment you have completed. Some treatments will put you at a higher risk for cardiovascular issues and even a return of the cancer, so be sure that you speak with your doctor and make plans to monitor the effects of your previous treatments.

240.   Understand that individuals who are battling cancer will need some time to themselves. Respect their wishes and do not force your presence on them if they need time to reflect and relax. You can also help by giving other visitors a signal to leave when your friend is getting tired.

241.   Mood swings and other similar symptoms are natural for those suffering from cancer. Knowing this can help you prepare for what you will encounter if you or a loved one are suffering with cancer.

242.   It is important for cancer patients to drink plenty of water, especially if they are receiving chemotherapy. A cancer patient's immune

system is low and it is important to stay hydrated. Becoming dehydrated can cause other complications that could land you in the hospital. Try to stay away from soda and sugary drinks.

243.   Protect your eyes from the sun! Be sure that the sunglasses that you buy are UV resistant. If you just buy any pair and do not check, the sun may not seem as bright but it is still doing the damage to the skin around your eyes and your eyes themselves.

244.   If you are 50 years or older, it is important that you get a colonoscopy at least once every 5 years. If you are at risk for colon cancer, it should be every two years. A colonoscopy can detect changes in the cells, and if treated early, can save your life.

245.   Stay organized. You are going to have many appointments to go to and have to keep track of many different dates. Get a calendar and use it to keep track of things that are important. You can even log how you have felt on different days so you can let your doctor in on your progress.

246.   You must quit smoking. Whether you have been diagnosed with cancer or you haven't yet been, smoking has to cease. This rule isn't just

for your lungs, it is for all parts of your body. Smoking is very harmful and contains carcinogenic chemicals which are detrimental to your body. Stop smoking!

247.   An easy way to avoid cancer is to not smoke. If you are already a smoker, it is never too late to quit. Even if you have tried to quit before, keep trying! Something will work eventually and it is better to keep trying than to keep puffing away.

248.   Watch out for cancer treatment scams. After being diagnosed with cancer, you may feel desperate to try any treatment you can find. However, you should be careful and fully research any treatment method you are considering. If a cancer "cure" sounds too good to be true, it probably is. Discuss and research the treatment with a reputable doctor or government agency before deciding on any treatment.

249.   One of the alternative treatments to cancer that you can add in addition to your doctors orders is a mind and body therapy. This therapy focuses on behavior, faith and emotions. The treatments can include hypnosis, biofeedback and counseling. These techniques will not cure

cancer but can greatly change your attitude about it and give your emotional life a lift.

250.   Some screenings can detect if there's cancer, others can find the problems and prevent the cancer. Time goes fast, and it is important to test yourself every now and again.

251.   As soon as you are diagnosed with cancer, you need to contact your insurance company to see what is covered and what isn't. Treatment can be extremely expensive, so you will want to know what is covered and what is not. Once you have this information, you should sit down and discuss it with your doctor. You two can then come up with a treatment plan that will work for you and your budget.

252.   If you are a woman, and breast cancer worries you. Then it is best to have been regular scheduled mammograms to make sure you are cancer free. Breast cancer is easily treated, and often successfully treated as long it's caught before the usual time by scheduling a routine mammogram you enable yourself to find out early enough to make a difference

253.   To reduce your risk for various types of cancers, not smoking or using tobacco in any

way is one of the best and easiest methods. Smoking has been linked not only to lunch cancer but also to lung, bladder, cervix and kidney cancer. Don't take the risk, and quit now, or don't start!

254.   One way to reduce your risk of cancer is to get immunized. Hepatitis B and HPV (human papillomavirus) can both lead to cancer. The Hep B vaccine is routinely given to infants, but is also recommended for adults who are considered at risk, such as people with multiple sexual partners or who are regularly exposed to blood.

255.   When battling cancer it is important for you to try to find humor somewhere. Many people fall into depression while they are battling cancer and do not even realize it. It is understandable for someone to feel depressed about the diagnosis but fighting is what helps save lives. Humor can be a great way to put up a fight.

256.   Recognize intellectually that your physical appearance will probably change after a cancer diagnosis. If you go into treatment anticipating that you will eventually look different, you will have a much better attitude when those changes actually take place. Talk to your doctor about

what to expect as you prepare to begin your journey.

257.   It feels like you're going through the sickness too if someone you love has cancer, but you have to stay healthy in order to be supportive. Those late nights at the hospital and skipped meals can take their toll on your health. You're no good to anyone if you're frail, tired and weak. Keep your health up.

258.   Certain types of fungus you eat can actually help you to prevent cancer, like the Maitake mushroom. According to research conducted by Dr. Well, a famous cancer physician and researcher, extract of the Maitake mushroom completely eliminated tumors in over 40% of all animals tested and shrunk tumor size in the other 60%.

259.   Communication is the key! If you feel the support from your friends and family is not sufficient, speak with them directly about this subject. Have a cordial conversation with them to let them know what they can do to help you and why you need help. But, go forward with your talk carefully. This is a challenging and emotional time. Try to make people act out of love. Live with no regrets.

260.   Eat at least 2 servings of blueberries a day. Studies have shown blueberries contain pterostilbene. Pterostilbene is said to help prevent colon-cancer. In addition, blueberries have Vitamin C. Large does of vitamin C have been linked to a decrease in oral lesions. Breakfast is a great time to include them in your diet.

261.   Make sure that you are up-to-date on your immunizations. Viral infections can have an impact on certain types of cancer so ask your doctor whether you have received all the necessary immunizations. In particular find out whether you have the Hepatitis B and HPV immunizations; these can help prevent liver cancer and cervical cancer.

262.   Wear a strong SPF protection sunscreen every day. This can help to reduce your risk of skin cancer. The sun emits damaging ultraviolet rays, but sunscreen can help to protect you from them. Look for a high quality sunscreen that contains both UVA and UVB protection for best results.

263.   Protect your eyes from the sun! Be sure that the sunglasses that you buy are UV resistant. If

you just buy any pair and do not check, the sun may not seem as bright but it is still doing the damage to the skin around your eyes and your eyes themselves.

264.   There are certain therapies that can assist you in treating your disease and helping you with life afterwards. Complementary therapies include massages, aromatherapy, acupuncture, and yoga. These are all ways to help you relax during one of the most stressful times in your life.

265.   If your cancer treatments are giving you diarrhea, try to eliminate the coffee that you may find so dear. Whilst the caffeine in coffee can make you feel more energized, it is also a diuretic which can make diarrhea worse. Along these lines, it is wise to discontinue use of all types of caffeine while in treatment to eliminate your diarrhea.

266.   You are going to find out who your true friends are during this time. Your true friends are going to be there to help when you are sick, take you to a movie when you are feeling great, make your meals when you cannot and just be there to listen as you complain about what you are going through.

267.   Avoiding cancer sounds like something that cannot be done, but by cutting things out of your life that increases the chances you are sure to have a better shot at avoiding the diagnosis. Avoiding all tobacco products is going to help you avoid it. If you have tried and failed try again until you succeed.

268.   Chemotherapy can damage the body in many ways. One key to remaining healthy throughout your treatment is to keep your weight stable and your immune system strong. If you are losing weight, eat calorie-rich, sugar-free foods. Also use foods and vitamins to boost your immune system, such as vitamin C, garlic and tomatoes.

269.   Alcohol consumption is the number one cause of liver cancer. Alcohol abuse over time can damage the liver in such a way that it can no longer function. Without a transplant, most liver cancers are fatal. Reduce your risk of liver cancer by cutting down your alcohol consumption or eliminating it completely.

270.   Ask your doctor plenty of questions. If you have just received a cancer diagnosis, make sure to get as much basic information as you can. Find out the type, if it can be treated, what the treatment would be, and if the cancer is

spreading. The more you know the better chance you will have.

271.   Always wash fruits and vegetables because they may contain traces of pesticides or harmful bacteria. Pesticides are used to prevent insects and other issues from causing destruction to the crops. Prior to consumptions, wash them with a mild soap to remove these pesticides or buy foods that have had minimal exposure to pesticides.

272.   Women who want to fight against breast cancer should understand how their breasts feel normally so that they can spot any change. Self-exams and paying close attention to the breasts is how you can accurately and immediately spot any change when you see or feel it. Many women are saved through self-exams.

273.   What you expect to have happen, and what actually happens, are two different things. Remember to thank those who support you for what they are able to do.

274.   Do not be fooled into believing that alcohol in any way helps to prevent cancer. Wine can prevent cancer because it contains grapes.

Ingesting a big amount of alcohol could place you at more risk in developing cancer.

275.   If you have been diagnosed with cancer, drink as much water as possible, ideally between eight and ten glasses every day. You will be taking quite a bit of medication, and water helps your kidneys handle everything that you are putting into your body. Water will also keep you hydrated.

276.   For cancer patients who are not satisfied with their current treatment, know that you can get a second opinion. Sometimes, another oncologist may know of treatment options that can help you. If you are unsure where to go for treatment, you can look online for good cancer treatment centers in your area.

277.   For people with moles on their bodies, be sure to always check for any changes, including an increase in size, a color change, or a change in shape. If you notice any of these changes, be sure to see a dermatologist immediately, as this could be a sign of skin cancer.

278.   For cancer patients in an extreme amount of pain, you may want to consider acupuncture. One of the many positive results of acupuncture

is that it helps to ease pain. There are even certain insurance companies who will cover acupuncture, if it is being used to manage pain from cancer.

279.	Know your family history. Once of the causes of skin cancer is genetics. If you have members in your family that have had skin cancer, you may be at more of a risk to get it as well. If you have inherited the traits of the high risk factor, you need to be additionally careful when in the sun.

280.	Beware that breast cancer can occur in women of all ages. Many women think that because they are in their twenties or thirties that they cannot get breast cancer, therefore, they ignore symptoms, like lumps in their breasts. If you feel anything suspicious, be sure to let your doctor know.

281.	If your cancer treatments are limiting your mobility, begin sleeping in a bedroom with easy access to a bathroom. You do not want to hurt yourself trying to get to a bathroom that is too far away or too difficult to enter. You may also want to consider making a few modifications to the bathroom, including installing a handrail.

282.   After cancer treatment, try to achieve and maintain your ideal weight. Many patients gain or lose weight during treatment, so take this process slowly and work with your doctor to reach your goal weight. Regardless of whether you have to gain or lose, be kind to your body throughout the process.

283.   Take time out of your schedule to pamper yourself a bit. You can go and get a manicure and pedicure or just take a candlelit bath. This time is important and you should really make the most out of every minute that you have to relax and enjoy time.

284.   Dealing with a devastating disease like cancer can cause many fears about life and death. A good way to help yourself overcome these feelings is to become more spiritual! Studies show that people who engage in regular worship and prayer fare much better and live longer than those who don't.

285.   After finding out that you have cancer, it is best to keep an open contact with your doctor and those close to you, such as your family members and close friends. If you avoid talking to them about your situation and your feelings, you might begin to feel isolated.

286.   Open up to others with cancer. You may feel that your friends and family, who have never had cancer, may not understand what you are going through. There are many support groups for those who have cancer or have survived cancer. There are also online message boards and forums where people speak candidly.

287.   People who suspect they may have cancer should rush to the doctor right away to get properly diagnosed. The earlier the cancer is caught in the body, the better your odds are of beating this terrible disease and living a normal life. Early stages of cancer can be defeated with therapy and/or surgery.

288.   Depression often causes health issues of its own, which can lead to problems treating the cancer. It's possible that they'll give up without even fighting back.

289.   Try limiting fat in your diet. By decreasing the amount of fat, you will lower your cancer risk. Avoid frying, especially deep frying. There are alternatives to frying such as baking, roasting, broiling, and steaming. Try to buy the low or non fat versions of your favorite foods, like milk and yogurt.

290.   The odds are great that your hair is going to fall out when you undergo chemotherapy, so you can initiate this process instead of being a victim to it. Shave your head in advance and you will reclaim the power here. You can make the choice instead of allowing chemo to make it for you.

291.   You're going to be running back and forth to the bathroom a lot as you fight with your cancer, so move into any bedroom that's closest to a bathroom. Being in close proximity to a bathroom will help to prevent accidents, and you also have quick and direct access to the shower when you need to freshen up.

292.   Always wear sunscreen. Taking this simple step can help reduce the risk of getting cancer from the sun. Try to stay in the shade as much as possible and also wear clothing and hats that will protect your skin. Apply sunscreen liberally and often to get the maximum amount of protection possible.

293.   In an effort to prevent cancer - stay away from tobacco products! This includes smoking and chewing tobacco. These items have been shown to increase the likelihood that you will develop lung, bladder, cervical, oral, and

pancreatic as well as kidney cancer. Avoiding them will not only help reduce your risk of cancer, it will help you lead a healthier lifestyle overall.

294.   Stay informed throughout your treatment process if you are currently dealing with cancer. The worst thing you could do is ignore your treatment or fail to care. You want to know what you are taking, what therapy you are doing, and how these things are intended to help treat your disease.

295.   Purchase mouthwash. Cancer treatment, including chemotherapy, will often cause you to form painful mouth ulcers. Mouthwash will help prevent these from occurring over time. Invest in a soft toothbrush as well, as regular tooth care can also impact the formation of mouth ulcers. These items will give you the added benefit of having fresh breath each day!

296.   Wear a strong SPF protection sunscreen every day. This can help to reduce your risk of skin cancer. The sun emits damaging ultraviolet rays, but sunscreen can help to protect you from them. Look for a high quality sunscreen that contains both UVA and UVB protection for best results.

297. Keep your babies out of the sun as much as possible. Use swim shirts when out at the beach or at the pool. Keep the sunscreen flowing and apply it to them quite often. Even if the sunscreen claims to be waterproof, they are sure to be losing some of the protection as they swim.

298. If you have beaten cancer, it is still important that you regularly see your doctor for checkups. Even it may be gone now, certain cancers can come back or they can begin in other parts of the body. If you notice any new symptoms, be sure to see your doctor right away.

299. A good tip for coping with a cancer diagnosis is to maintain a healthy lifestyle. A healthy diet, plenty of rest, and physical activity are all important for staying healthy. Staying fit will give you the stamina you need to battle cancer, as well as the ability to bounce back after your treatment.

300. While you have cancer it is of dire importance that you keep yourself healthy. The best way to do this is by protecting yourself from germs. The best way is to stay on top of germs by using a disinfectant on every surface others

touch. Be especially mindful of things such as door knobs, toilets, sinks, and telephones.

301.   Install a panic button of some kind in your bathroom. You are going to need to shower regularly and there are going to be days that you are weaker than others. If you find yourself in the position that you need help, you need to be able to alert someone that you need that help.

302.   Focus on having a healthy diet during your cancer treatment. Eating better will give you more energy for everything that you are going through. It will also help you feel less stressed because your body will have the fuel it needs for the day. Research has shown that eating well may also extend your life.

303.   When it is necessary you should speak up. A lot of people still have old fashioned beliefs about cancer, and some even believe that cancer can be transmitted from person to person. By thinking about these answers in advance, you will be better prepared when these questions arise. This way, others who are around you will be in a better position to support you during treatment, as their fears will have been allayed.

304.   Many people think that smoking only causes emphysema and lung cancer; however, smoking also causes colon cancer. Tobacco smoke has cancer-causing agents that get into the colon, and it can also make colon polyps much bigger. All of these concerns add up to serious reasons to put aside those cigarettes for good.

305.   Expressing your love for someone with cancer doesn't always have to be done vocally. You can simply be there for a person physically to assist them and to show your moral support. Some types of cancer are incredibly rough, and the patient might not be able to care for him or herself. Make sure you're there for them.

306.   Simple carbohydrates can actually increase your risk of getting cancer, but complex carbs, like whole grains, will reduce your risk significantly. The germ, bran and endosperm of the whole grains are very rich in fiber, vitamins and minerals and can help you to prevent cancer in your stomach, colon and other areas of the body.

307.   Decrease the amount of red (such as lamb, pork, and beef) and processed meats in your diet. Studies have shown that red meat can increase your chances of getting cancer. If you do buy red

meat, make sure that it is lean meat. You don't have to remove red meat from your diet, just limit it.

308.   Be open and honest with others. If you need additional help to get through this difficult period in your life, bring the topic up gently with your loved ones. Let them know how and why they can assist you. However, be sure to approach this topic gently. Approach this as a challenge. Make requests from a place of love, though. Do not live your life with regrets.

309.   Try to tone down the amount of time you spend in the sun. People underestimate the amount of risk involved with excessive sun exposure. Spending increased time in the sun increases your risk of skin cancer. Make sure to use a high SPF sunscreen, cover unprotected skin and cover your head with a hat.

310.   Offer to help with the daily chores or activities of someone with cancer. Treatment can be an exhausting process, but by simply making a dinner or doing someone's laundry is a gift that they will appreciate immensely. Don't just make a vague offer to help, give them a specific day and time that you will come over.

311.   Take vitamin E on a daily basis. Vitamin E in its recommended daily dose has been found to have profound effects in preventing cancer in men and women. Plenty of foods contain enough vitamin E for you to get your daily dosage.

312.   Get to know your breasts. It may seem kind of silly to feel your breasts on a regular basis, but if you take the time to learn how they should feel, you are going to be able to notice any changes if they should occur. This makes it much easier for you to know when there is a change so you can see your doctor immediately.

313.   Before you begin chemotherapy treatment, it may be wise to shave your head. As many people know, chemotherapy makes your hair fall out. What people do not know is that it does not all come out at once; it comes out in bunches. Shaving your head will prevent you from having hair in some spots but not others.

314.   Be aware of, and monitor, your body's signals for what it needs. If your energy is low, then take a break. A diet change to a healthier diet might help fight that feeling of fatigue. Heed the advice your body gives you in the form of malaise.

315.   Keep a telephone within an arm's reach of your bed. While you are undergoing cancer treatments, there may be times when you need immediate assistance. Having a phone close by will give you the opportunity to get help if you need it. This also makes it easy for you to call friends and family members to chat.

316.   Seek help from your religious leader. If you do not have one, there are many that will be more than happy to help you through this time. If you are looking for someone to pray with you or just to listen without judgment, they are going to be what you need.

317.   If you have a loved one that is experiencing cancer, a good way to encourage them is to go with them on their appointments. Attending appointments will let them know that you love and care for them. Hospitals and clinics can be frightening to some people, and waiting long hours can be really boring. With that said, having a companion is really a big deal.